30 DIY COSMETIC PRODUCTS THAT

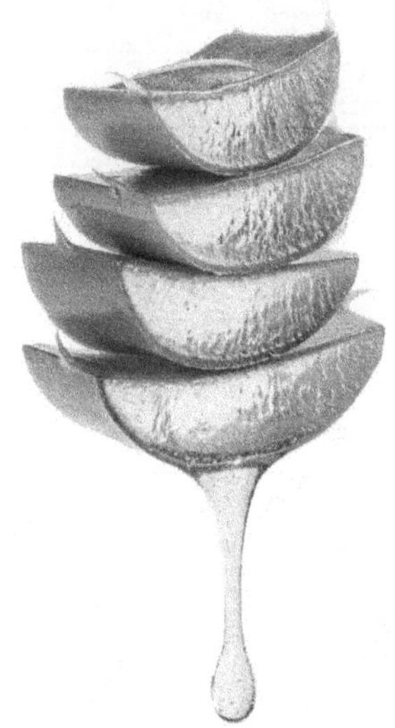

CAN BE MADE FROM ALOE VERA GEL

BY CHARLES OBINJU

Introduction

Aloe vera, known for its soothing and healing properties, is a versatile plant that can be used in a wide range of DIY products. From skincare to haircare, aloe vera gel serves as a natural and nourishing ingredient that can be incorporated into various homemade creations. Whether you're looking to make a refreshing face mask, a moisturizing lotion, a cooling spray, or a nourishing hair conditioner, aloe vera DIY products offer a fantastic way to harness the benefits of this plant and create personalized, natural solutions for your beauty and wellness routine. With a few simple ingredients and a little creativity, you can tap into the power of aloe vera to enhance your self-care rituals and indulge in the numerous benefits it has to offer.

Aloe vera Extraction

Extracting aloe vera gel from an aloe vera plant is a simple process that can be done at home. Here's a step-by-step guide to extracting aloe vera gel:

Select a mature aloe vera leaf: Choose a thick and healthy leaf from an aloe vera plant that is at least a couple of years old. The larger, outer leaves tend to contain more gel. Prepare the leaf: Carefully cut or snap off the selected leaf from the base of the plant. Rinse the leaf under cool water to remove any dirt or debris.

Allow the yellow resin to drain: After rinsing, place the leaf upright in a container or on a cutting board with the cut end facing downward. This position allows the yellow resin, known as aloin, to drain out. Aloin can cause skin irritation and has a bitter taste, so it's important to let it drain.

Slice the leaf: Once the resin has drained, use a clean, sharp knife to cut off the spiky edges of the leaf. Then make a lengthwise incision along one side of the leaf to expose the gel inside.

Scoop out the gel: With the leaf open, use a spoon or your fingers to gently scoop out the translucent gel from the leaf. Place the extracted gel into a clean bowl or container. Be careful not to scrape the yellow resin from the leaf, as it can mix with the gel.

Store the gel: Once you have extracted all the gel, transfer it to an airtight container for storage. You can refrigerate the gel to prolong its shelf life and enhance its cooling effect.

Soothing Aloe Vera Face Mask:

To create a soothing aloe vera face mask, you'll need a few simple ingredients. Here's a recipe to make one:

Ingredients:

- 2 tablespoons of aloe vera gel
- 1 tablespoon of honey

Instructions:

- In a small bowl, combine the aloe vera gel and honey.
- Stir the mixture well until you have a smooth and consistent paste.
- Cleanse your face thoroughly to remove any dirt or makeup.
- Apply the aloe vera and honey mixture evenly to your face, avoiding the eye area.
- Leave the mask on for about 15-20 minutes to allow it to work its magic.
- Rinse your face with lukewarm water and pat dry with a clean towel.
- Follow up with your regular skincare routine, such as moisturizer or serum.

Benefits:

- Aloe vera gel has soothing properties that can help calm and hydrate the skin. It may also help reduce redness and inflammation.
- Honey is a natural humectant, meaning it helps retain moisture in the skin, leaving it soft and supple. It also has antibacterial properties that can benefit acne-prone skin.

Note: If you have any known allergies to aloe vera or honey, it's important to avoid using this mask or do a patch test on a small area of your skin first to ensure you don't experience any adverse reactions.

Cooling Aloe Vera Sunburn Relief Gel:

To create a cooling aloe vera sunburn relief gel, you'll need aloe vera gel and a few additional ingredients for added soothing and cooling effects. Here's a simple recipe:

Ingredients:

- 1/4 cup of aloe vera gel
- 2-3 drops of lavender essential oil
- 2-3 drops of peppermint essential oil

Instructions:

- In a small bowl, combine the aloe vera gel, lavender essential oil, and peppermint essential oil.
- Mix the ingredients well until they are thoroughly blended.
- Transfer the mixture to a clean container with a lid for storage.

How to use:

- Cleanse the sunburned area gently with cool water and pat dry with a clean towel.
- Take a small amount of the cooling aloe vera gel and apply it directly to the sunburned skin.

- Gently massage the gel into the skin until it is absorbed.
- Repeat the application 2-3 times a day or as needed for relief.

Benefits:

- Aloe vera gel provides soothing and moisturizing properties, helping to alleviate sunburn discomfort and promote skin healing.
- Lavender essential oil has calming and anti-inflammatory properties that can further soothe the skin and reduce redness.
- Peppermint essential oil has a cooling sensation that can provide immediate relief from sunburn pain and inflammation.

Note: It's important to ensure that your sunburn is not severe or blistering. If you have a severe sunburn or experience any adverse reactions, it's recommended to consult a healthcare professional for proper treatment.

Refreshing Aloe Vera Facial Toner

Creating a refreshing aloe vera facial toner is a simple process that can help balance your skin's pH, tighten pores, and provide a refreshing boost. Here's a recipe to make your own aloe vera facial toner:

Ingredients:

- 1/2 cup of aloe vera gel
- 1/4 cup of witch hazel
- 1/4 cup of rose water

Instructions:

- In a clean container, combine the aloe vera gel, witch hazel, and rose water.
- Stir the mixture well to ensure the ingredients are thoroughly blended.
- Transfer the toner to a spray bottle or airtight container for convenient use.

How to use:

- Cleanse your face with a gentle cleanser and pat dry.
- Close your eyes and spray the aloe vera facial toner directly onto your face, or apply it using a cotton pad.
- Gently press the toner into your skin, allowing it to absorb.
- Follow up with your regular moisturizer or serum.

Benefits:

- Aloe vera gel helps hydrate and soothe the skin, making it an excellent ingredient for toners.
- Witch hazel is a natural astringent that can help tighten pores and reduce excess oil production.
- Rose water has refreshing and toning properties, leaving the skin feeling revitalized.

Note: It's always recommended to do a patch test before using any new product on your face, especially if you have sensitive skin, to ensure you don't have any adverse reactions.

Nourishing Aloe Vera Hair Mask:

Creating a nourishing aloe vera hair mask is a great way to promote healthy hair and provide deep hydration. Here's a simple recipe for a DIY aloe vera hair mask:

Ingredients:
- 1/2 cup of aloe vera gel
- 2 tablespoons of coconut oil
- 1 tablespoon of honey
- Optional: a few drops of essential oil for fragrance (such as lavender or rosemary)

Instructions:
- In a mixing bowl, combine the aloe vera gel, coconut oil, and honey.
- If desired, add a few drops of your chosen essential oil for a pleasant fragrance.
- Mix the ingredients well until they form a smooth and consistent mixture.
- Start with dry or slightly damp hair. Divide your hair into sections to make the application easier.
- Take a generous amount of the aloe vera hair mask and apply it from the roots to the ends of your hair, ensuring it is evenly distributed.
- Gently massage the mask into your scalp to promote blood circulation.
- Once your hair is completely coated, cover it with a shower cap or wrap it in a towel.
- Leave the hair mask on for 30 minutes to 1 hour to allow the ingredients to penetrate and nourish your hair.
- After the recommended time, rinse your hair thoroughly with lukewarm water.
- Follow up with your regular shampoo and conditioner routine.

Benefits:
- Aloe vera gel helps hydrate the hair, improve its elasticity, and reduce frizz.
- Coconut oil is deeply moisturizing and nourishing for the hair, helping to strengthen and prevent breakage.
- Honey acts as a natural humectant, locking in moisture and promoting softness and shine.

Note: Adjust the quantities of the ingredients based on your hair length and thickness. If you have any known allergies to the ingredients, it's important to avoid using this mask or do a patch test on a small area of your skin first to ensure you don't experience any adverse reactions.

Moisturizing Aloe Vera Body Lotion:

Creating a moisturizing aloe vera body lotion is a fantastic way to hydrate and nourish your skin. Here's a recipe for a DIY aloe vera body lotion:

Ingredients:
- 1/2 cup of aloe vera gel
- 1/4 cup of shea butter
- 2 tablespoons of almond oil

- Optional: a few drops of your preferred essential oil for fragrance (such as lavender or vanilla)

Instructions:

- In a double boiler or a heat-safe bowl placed over a pot of simmering water, melt the shea butter until it becomes liquid.
- Remove the melted shea butter from the heat and allow it to cool slightly.
- Add the almond oil to the melted shea butter and mix well.
- Let the mixture cool further until it reaches room temperature.
- In a separate bowl, combine the aloe vera gel and the cooled shea butter and almond oil mixture.
- If desired, add a few drops of your chosen essential oil for a pleasant fragrance.
- Using a hand mixer or a blender, whip the ingredients together until they are well blended and reach a creamy consistency.
- Transfer the lotion to a clean and airtight container for storage.

How to use:

- Take a small amount of the aloe vera body lotion and apply it to your skin.
- Gently massage the lotion into your skin, focusing on dry areas or areas that need extra hydration.
- Allow the lotion to absorb fully before dressing.

Benefits:

- Aloe vera gel is known for its soothing and moisturizing properties, which can help hydrate and soften the skin.
- Shea butter is deeply nourishing and can provide long-lasting moisturization.
- Almond oil is rich in vitamins and fatty acids, helping to moisturize and improve the overall appearance of the skin.

Note: If you have any known allergies to the ingredients, it's important to avoid using this lotion or do a patch test on a small area of your skin first to ensure you don't experience any adverse reactions.

Aloe Vera Shaving Gel:

Creating a homemade aloe vera shaving gel is a great alternative to commercial shaving creams that can be harsh on the skin. Here's a simple recipe for a DIY aloe vera shaving gel:

Ingredients:

- 1/4 cup of aloe vera gel
- 1/4 cup of liquid castile soap (unscented or your preferred fragrance)
- 1 tablespoon of almond oil or coconut oil
- Optional: a few drops of essential oil for fragrance (such as peppermint or lavender)

Instructions:

In a bowl, combine the aloe vera gel, liquid castile soap, and almond oil (or coconut oil). If desired, add a few drops of your chosen essential oil for a pleasant fragrance and additional benefits.

Stir the ingredients together until they are well blended.

Transfer the shaving gel to a clean and airtight container for storage.

How to use:

Wet the area you want to shave with warm water to soften the hair and prepare the skin.

Take a small amount of the aloe vera shaving gel and apply it to the area.

Use your hands or a shaving brush to work the gel into a lather.

Shave as usual, rinsing the blade frequently to prevent clogging.

After shaving, rinse the area thoroughly with water and pat dry.

Benefits:

- Aloe vera gel helps provide a smooth and lubricating surface for the razor, reducing the risk of irritation and razor burn.
- Liquid castile soap creates a light lather that helps the razor glide easily over the skin.
- Almond oil or coconut oil adds moisture and nourishment to the skin, leaving it feeling soft and smooth.

Note: Adjust the quantities of the ingredients based on your preference and the size of the container you are using. If you have any known allergies to the ingredients, it's important to avoid using this shaving gel or do a patch test on a small area of your skin first to ensure you don't experience any adverse reactions.

Aloe Vera Gel for Acne:

Aloe vera gel can be a beneficial natural remedy for acne due to its soothing and anti-inflammatory properties. Here's how you can use aloe vera gel for acne:

- Cleanse your face: Start by cleansing your face with a gentle cleanser to remove dirt, excess oil, and makeup. Pat dry with a clean towel.
- Extract fresh aloe vera gel: If you have an aloe vera plant, cut a leaf and extract the gel by slicing it open lengthwise. Scoop out the gel with a spoon. If you don't have a plant, you can use store-bought aloe vera gel, just make sure it is pure and free of any added chemicals or fragrances.
- Apply a thin layer of aloe vera gel: Take a small amount of aloe vera gel and apply a thin layer to the affected areas of your skin. Gently massage it in using circular motions.
- Leave it on: Allow the aloe vera gel to dry on your skin. There is no need to rinse it off, as it can be left on as a moisturizer.
- Repeat daily: For best results, apply aloe vera gel to your acne-prone skin twice a day, once in the morning and once in the evening.

Benefits of using aloe vera gel for acne:

- Aloe vera gel has anti-inflammatory properties that can help reduce redness, swelling, and inflammation associated with acne.
- It has soothing properties that can alleviate the discomfort and irritation caused by acne.
- Aloe vera gel can moisturize the skin without clogging pores, as it is lightweight and non-greasy.
- It may help promote healing and reduce the appearance of acne scars over time.

Note: Although aloe vera gel is generally considered safe for most skin types, it's always a good idea to do a patch test on a small area of your skin first to ensure you don't have any adverse reactions. If you experience any irritation or discomfort, discontinue use. If your acne is severe or persistent, it's recommended to consult a dermatologist for appropriate treatment.

Aloe Vera Gel Hand Sanitizer:

Creating a homemade aloe vera gel hand sanitizer is a useful option when commercial sanitizers are not readily available. Here's a simple recipe for a DIY aloe vera gel hand sanitizer:

Ingredients:

- 2/3 cup of isopropyl alcohol (99% or at least 70% concentration)
- 1/3 cup of aloe vera gel
- Optional: a few drops of essential oil for fragrance (such as tea tree oil or lavender oil)

Instructions:

- In a bowl, combine the isopropyl alcohol and aloe vera gel.
- If desired, add a few drops of your chosen essential oil for a pleasant fragrance and additional antimicrobial properties.
- Stir the mixture well until all ingredients are thoroughly blended.
- Pour the hand sanitizer into a clean and airtight container for storage.

How to use:

- Apply a small amount of the hand sanitizer to the palm of one hand.
- Rub your hands together, ensuring you cover all surfaces of your hands and fingers.
- Continue rubbing for about 20-30 seconds or until the sanitizer has evaporated and your hands feel dry.

Important considerations:

- The alcohol content is crucial for an effective hand sanitizer. Make sure you use isopropyl alcohol with a concentration of at least 70%.
- Aloe vera gel is added to the recipe to help moisturize and soothe the skin, as alcohol can be drying. It also helps create a gel-like consistency.
- Essential oils, such as tea tree oil, can provide additional antimicrobial properties, but be cautious with the amount used, as some essential oils may cause skin irritation in high concentrations.

Note: Hand sanitizers are not a substitute for thorough handwashing with soap and water, especially when hands are visibly dirty or greasy. Additionally, this homemade hand sanitizer may not be as effective as commercial ones, so it's recommended to use it when soap and water are not available.

Aloe Vera Gel Makeup Remover

Aloe vera gel can be a gentle and effective option for removing makeup. Here's how you can use aloe vera gel as a makeup remover:

- Gather the necessary supplies: You will need pure aloe vera gel and cotton pads or a clean, soft cloth.
- Extract fresh aloe vera gel: If you have an aloe vera plant, cut a leaf and extract the gel by slicing it open lengthwise. Scoop out the gel with a spoon. If you don't have a plant, you can use store-bought pure aloe vera gel.
- Apply aloe vera gel to the cotton pad or cloth: Take a small amount of aloe vera gel and apply it to a cotton pad or a clean, soft cloth. You can use more or less depending on the amount of makeup you need to remove.
- Gently cleanse the face: Start by closing your eyes and placing the aloe vera gel-soaked cotton pad or cloth over your eyelids for a few seconds to allow the makeup to dissolve. Then, gently wipe the cotton pad or cloth over your face, including the eye area, lips, and any other areas with makeup. Be gentle and avoid rubbing too vigorously, especially around the delicate eye area.
- Repeat if necessary: If there is still residual makeup, repeat the process using a fresh cotton pad or cloth with aloe vera gel until your face is clean and makeup-free.
- Rinse or moisturize: After removing the makeup, you can rinse your face with water to remove any remaining aloe vera gel or simply proceed with your regular skincare routine. If you prefer, you can also apply a moisturizer or toner after using the aloe vera gel as a makeup remover.

Benefits of using aloe vera gel as a makeup remover:

- Aloe vera gel is gentle on the skin and suitable for all skin types, including sensitive skin.
- It helps dissolve and lift makeup, including waterproof products, without harsh chemicals or drying ingredients.
- Aloe vera gel is moisturizing and can help soothe and hydrate the skin, leaving it feeling refreshed.

Note: If you have any known allergies to aloe vera gel, it's important to avoid using it as a makeup remover or do a patch test on a small area of your skin first to ensure you don't experience any adverse reactions.

Aloe Vera Gel Makeup Remover:

Aloe vera gel can be a gentle and effective makeup remover, suitable for all skin types. Here's a simple method to use aloe vera gel as a makeup remover:

- Gather the necessary supplies: You will need pure aloe vera gel, cotton pads, and a clean towel.
- Extract fresh aloe vera gel: If you have an aloe vera plant, cut a leaf and extract the gel by slicing it open lengthwise. Scoop out the gel with a spoon. If you don't have a plant, you can use store-bought pure aloe vera gel.

- Apply aloe vera gel to a cotton pad: Take a cotton pad and apply a small amount of aloe vera gel to it. You can use more or less depending on the amount of makeup you need to remove.
- Gently wipe away makeup: Close your eyes and place the aloe vera gel-soaked cotton pad on your eyelids for a few seconds to allow the makeup to loosen. Then, starting with your eyes, gently wipe the cotton pad over your face, focusing on areas with makeup. Continue wiping until the makeup is effectively removed. Be gentle and avoid rubbing too harshly, especially around the eye area.
- Rinse or cleanse: After removing the makeup with the aloe vera gel, you can rinse your face with water to remove any residue. Alternatively, you can follow up with your regular facial cleanser to cleanse the skin thoroughly.
- Pat dry and moisturize: Once your face is clean, pat it dry with a clean towel. Follow up with your preferred moisturizer to hydrate and nourish your skin.

Benefits of using aloe vera gel as a makeup remover:
- Aloe vera gel is gentle and suitable for sensitive skin, reducing the risk of irritation or allergic reactions.
- It effectively breaks down and removes makeup, including waterproof formulas.
- Aloe vera gel has moisturizing properties that can leave your skin feeling hydrated and refreshed.
- It can help soothe and calm the skin, reducing redness and inflammation caused by makeup removal.

Note: If you have any known allergies to aloe vera gel, it's important to avoid using it as a makeup remover or do a patch test on a small area of your skin first to ensure you don't experience any adverse reactions.

Aloe Vera Lip Balm:

Making your own aloe vera lip balm is a great way to keep your lips moisturized and nourished. Here's a simple recipe for DIY aloe vera lip balm:

Ingredients:
- 1 tablespoon of pure aloe vera gel
- 1 tablespoon of coconut oil
- 1 teaspoon of beeswax pellets
- Optional: a few drops of your preferred essential oil for fragrance (such as peppermint or lavender)

Instructions:
- In a double boiler or a heat-safe bowl placed over a pot of simmering water, melt the coconut oil and beeswax pellets together.
- Stir the mixture until the beeswax is fully melted and the ingredients are well combined.
- Remove the mixture from heat and let it cool for a few minutes.
- Add the aloe vera gel to the melted coconut oil and beeswax mixture.
- If desired, add a few drops of your chosen essential oil for a pleasant fragrance.

- Stir well to ensure all ingredients are thoroughly blended.
- Pour the mixture into small lip balm containers or empty lip balm tubes.
- Let the lip balm cool and solidify completely before using.

How to use:

- Apply the aloe vera lip balm to your lips as needed throughout the day.
- Reapply whenever your lips feel dry or in need of moisture.

Benefits:

- Aloe vera gel provides hydration and soothing properties to help alleviate dryness and chapped lips.
- Coconut oil is deeply moisturizing and helps create a protective barrier on the lips to retain moisture.
- Beeswax provides a solidifying agent, giving the lip balm a solid texture and making it convenient for application.

Note: Adjust the quantities of the ingredients based on the number of lip balm containers you wish to fill. If you have any known allergies to the ingredients, it's important to avoid using this lip balm or do a patch test on a small area of your skin first to ensure you don't experience any adverse reactions.

Aloe Vera Gel Hair Gel:

Creating a DIY aloe vera gel hair gel is a natural and nourishing way to style and manage your hair. Here's a simple recipe to make aloe vera gel hair gel:

Ingredients:

- 1/2 cup of aloe vera gel
- 1 teaspoon of coconut oil or argan oil (optional)
- 1-2 drops of your preferred essential oil for fragrance (optional)

Instructions:

- In a bowl, combine the aloe vera gel and coconut oil or argan oil.
- If desired, add a few drops of your chosen essential oil for a pleasant fragrance.
- Mix the ingredients well until they are thoroughly blended.
- Transfer the mixture to a clean and airtight container for storage.

How to use:

- Start with clean, damp hair.
- Take a small amount of the aloe vera gel hair gel and rub it between your palms to warm it up.
- Apply the gel evenly throughout your hair, focusing on the roots and working your way to the ends.
- Style your hair as desired using your fingers or a comb.
- Let your hair air dry or use a diffuser for a defined look.

Benefits:

- Aloe vera gel helps provide hold and definition to your hair without leaving it stiff or crunchy.

- Coconut oil or argan oil can add moisture and shine to your hair, making it more manageable and reducing frizz.
- Essential oils can provide a pleasant scent and some additional benefits for the hair and scalp, depending on the chosen oil.

Note: Adjust the quantities of the ingredients based on the length and thickness of your hair. If you have any known allergies to the ingredients, it's important to avoid using this hair gel or do a patch test on a small area of your skin first to ensure you don't experience any adverse reactions.

Aloe Vera Gel Foot Scrub:

Aloe vera gel can be a soothing and moisturizing ingredient in a homemade foot scrub. Here's a simple recipe for a DIY aloe vera gel foot scrub:

Ingredients:
- 1/2 cup of granulated sugar or sea salt
- 2 tablespoons of aloe vera gel
- 2 tablespoons of coconut oil or olive oil
- Optional: a few drops of essential oil for fragrance (such as peppermint or lavender)

Instructions:
- In a bowl, combine the granulated sugar or sea salt with the aloe vera gel and coconut oil or olive oil.
- If desired, add a few drops of your chosen essential oil for a pleasant fragrance and added benefits.
- Mix all the ingredients together until well combined, creating a thick and gritty paste.

How to use:
- Soak your feet in warm water for a few minutes to soften the skin.
- Take a small amount of the aloe vera gel foot scrub and apply it to one foot, focusing on the rough areas like heels and calluses.
- Gently massage the scrub into your foot using circular motions, paying attention to exfoliate and remove dead skin cells.
- Repeat the process on the other foot.
- Rinse your feet with warm water to remove the scrub.
- Pat your feet dry with a clean towel.
- Apply a moisturizer or foot cream to nourish and hydrate your feet.

Benefits:
- Aloe vera gel helps soothe and moisturize the skin on your feet, leaving them soft and hydrated.
- Granulated sugar or sea salt act as natural exfoliants to remove dead skin cells and reveal smoother skin.
- Coconut oil or olive oil provide additional moisture and nourishment to your feet.

Note: Avoid using the foot scrub on any open wounds, cuts, or sensitive areas of the feet. If you have any known allergies to the ingredients, it's important to avoid using this foot scrub or do a patch test on a small area of your skin first to ensure you don't experience any adverse reactions.

Aloe Vera Gel Body Wash:

Creating your own aloe vera gel body wash is a wonderful way to cleanse and nourish your skin. Here's a simple recipe for a DIY aloe vera gel body wash:

Ingredients:

- 1 cup of unscented liquid castile soap
- 1/4 cup of aloe vera gel
- 1 tablespoon of sweet almond oil or jojoba oil
- Optional: a few drops of your preferred essential oil for fragrance (such as lavender or citrus)

Instructions:

- In a bowl, combine the unscented liquid castile soap, aloe vera gel, and sweet almond oil or jojoba oil.
- If desired, add a few drops of your chosen essential oil for a pleasant scent and additional benefits.
- Stir all the ingredients together until well blended.
- Pour the mixture into a clean, empty bottle or dispenser for storage.

How to use:

- In the shower or bath, wet your body.
- Take a small amount of the aloe vera gel body wash in your hand or onto a loofah or washcloth.
- Gently massage the body wash onto your skin, working it into a lather.
- Rinse off thoroughly with warm water.
- Follow with your favorite moisturizer if needed.

Benefits:

- Aloe vera gel helps moisturize and soothe the skin, leaving it feeling refreshed and hydrated.
- Liquid castile soap provides gentle cleansing without harsh ingredients or chemicals.
- Sweet almond oil or jojoba oil nourish and moisturize the skin, preventing dryness.

Note: If you have any known allergies to the ingredients, it's important to avoid using this body wash or do a patch test on a small area of your skin first to ensure you don't experience any adverse reactions. Additionally, be cautious with the amount of essential oil used, as some essential oils may cause skin irritation in high concentrations.

Aloe Vera Gel Body Wash:

Creating your own aloe vera gel body wash is a wonderful way to cleanse and nourish your skin. Here's a simple recipe for a DIY aloe vera gel body wash:

Ingredients:
- 1 cup of liquid castile soap (unscented or a mild, natural scent)
- 1/4 cup of aloe vera gel
- 1 tablespoon of sweet almond oil or jojoba oil
- Optional: a few drops of your preferred essential oil for fragrance (such as lavender or citrus)

Instructions:
- In a mixing bowl, combine the liquid castile soap, aloe vera gel, and sweet almond oil or jojoba oil.
- If desired, add a few drops of your chosen essential oil for a pleasant fragrance and added benefits.
- Stir all the ingredients together until well blended.
- Transfer the mixture to a clean, empty bottle or dispenser for storage.
- How to use:
- In the shower or bath, wet your body.
- Take a small amount of the aloe vera gel body wash in your hand or on a washcloth or loofah.
- Gently massage the body wash onto your skin, working it into a lather.
- Rinse off thoroughly with warm water.
- Follow with your favorite moisturizer if needed.

Benefits:
- Aloe vera gel helps moisturize and soothe the skin, leaving it feeling refreshed and hydrated.
- Liquid castile soap provides gentle cleansing without harsh ingredients or chemicals.
- Sweet almond oil or jojoba oil nourish and moisturize the skin, preventing dryness.
- Essential oils can add a pleasant scent and provide additional benefits for the skin, depending on the chosen oil.

Note: It's important to be cautious with the amount of essential oil used, as some essential oils may cause skin irritation in high concentrations. If you have any known allergies to the ingredients, it's important to avoid using this body wash or do a patch test on a small area of your skin first to ensure you don't experience any adverse reactions.

Aloe Vera Gel Body Wash:

Creating your own aloe vera gel body wash is a fantastic way to cleanse and nourish your skin. Here's a simple recipe for a DIY aloe vera gel body wash:

Ingredients:

- 1 cup of liquid castile soap (unscented or a mild, natural scent)
- 1/4 cup of aloe vera gel
- 1 tablespoon of vegetable glycerin
- Optional: a few drops of your preferred essential oil for fragrance (such as lavender or tea tree)

Instructions:

- In a mixing bowl, combine the liquid castile soap, aloe vera gel, and vegetable glycerin.
- If desired, add a few drops of your chosen essential oil for a pleasant scent and added benefits.
- Stir all the ingredients together until well blended.
- Transfer the mixture to a clean, empty bottle or dispenser for storage.

How to use:

- In the shower or bath, wet your body.
- Take a small amount of the aloe vera gel body wash in your hand or on a washcloth.
- Gently massage the body wash onto your skin, working it into a lather.
- Rinse off thoroughly with warm water.
- Follow with your favorite moisturizer if needed.

Benefits:

- Aloe vera gel helps moisturize and soothe the skin, leaving it feeling refreshed and hydrated.
- Liquid castile soap provides gentle cleansing without harsh ingredients or chemicals.
- Vegetable glycerin acts as a humectant, attracting and retaining moisture in the skin.
- Essential oils can add a pleasant scent and provide additional benefits for the skin, depending on the chosen oil.

Note: It's important to be cautious with the amount of essential oil used, as some essential oils may cause skin irritation in high concentrations. If you have any known allergies to the ingredients, it's important to avoid using this body wash or do a patch test on a small area of your skin first to ensure you don't experience any adverse reactions.

Aloe Vera Gel Eye Cream

Creating your own aloe vera gel eye cream is a wonderful way to hydrate and nourish the delicate skin around your eyes. Here's a simple recipe for a DIY aloe vera gel eye cream:

Ingredients:

- 2 tablespoons of pure aloe vera gel
- 1 tablespoon of sweet almond oil or coconut oil
- 1 teaspoon of vitamin E oil
- Optional: a few drops of rosehip oil or lavender essential oil

Instructions:

- In a small bowl, combine the pure aloe vera gel, sweet almond oil or coconut oil, and vitamin E oil.
- If desired, add a few drops of rosehip oil or lavender essential oil for added benefits and fragrance.
- Mix all the ingredients well until they are thoroughly combined.
- Transfer the mixture to a clean, airtight container for storage.

How to use:

- Cleanse your face and gently pat your eye area dry.
- Take a small amount of the aloe vera gel eye cream and dot it around your eye area.
- Using your ring finger, gently tap and massage the eye cream into the skin.
- Continue to massage until the eye cream is fully absorbed.
- Use the eye cream in the morning and evening as part of your skincare routine.

Benefits:

- Aloe vera gel hydrates and soothes the delicate skin around the eyes, reducing puffiness and dryness.
- Sweet almond oil or coconut oil nourishes and moisturizes the skin, improving its texture and elasticity.
- Vitamin E oil provides antioxidant properties, helping to protect the skin from environmental damage.
- Rosehip oil or lavender essential oil can offer additional benefits, such as reducing dark circles or calming the skin.

Note: If you have any known allergies to the ingredients, it's important to avoid using this eye cream or do a patch test on a small area of your skin first to ensure you don't experience any adverse reactions. Be careful not to get the eye cream into your eyes, as it is intended for external use only.

Aloe Vera Gel Makeup Setting Spray:

Making your own aloe vera gel makeup setting spray is a great way to keep your makeup in place and give your skin a refreshing boost. Here's a simple recipe for a DIY aloe vera gel makeup setting spray:

Ingredients:

- 1/4 cup of pure aloe vera gel
- 1/4 cup of distilled water
- 1 teaspoon of vegetable glycerin
- Optional: a few drops of your preferred essential oil for fragrance (such as rose or cucumber)

Instructions:

- In a small spray bottle, combine the pure aloe vera gel, distilled water, and vegetable glycerin.
- If desired, add a few drops of your chosen essential oil for a pleasant scent.
- Screw the spray bottle cap tightly and shake well to thoroughly mix all the ingredients.

How to use:

- Shake the bottle before each use to ensure the ingredients are well mixed.
- Hold the spray bottle about 6-8 inches away from your face.
- Close your eyes and mist the setting spray evenly over your face, keeping your mouth and eyes closed.
- Allow the setting spray to air dry and set your makeup.
- You can also use the setting spray throughout the day to refresh your makeup or provide a hydration boost to your skin.

Benefits:

- Aloe vera gel helps to set your makeup and keep it in place, while also soothing and hydrating the skin.
- Distilled water provides a base for the spray and adds moisture without any impurities.
- Vegetable glycerin acts as a humectant, helping to lock in moisture and prevent your makeup from looking dry or cakey.
- Essential oils can provide a pleasant fragrance and offer additional benefits, depending on the chosen oil.

Note: If you have any known allergies to the ingredients, it's important to avoid using this makeup setting spray or do a patch test on a small area of your skin first to ensure you don't experience any adverse reactions. Keep the spray bottle tightly closed when not in use to maintain the freshness and effectiveness of the product.

Aloe Vera Gel Cuticle Oil:

Creating your own aloe vera gel cuticle oil is a great way to nourish and moisturize your cuticles. Here's a simple recipe for a DIY aloe vera gel cuticle oil:

Ingredients:

- 1 tablespoon of pure aloe vera gel
- 1 tablespoon of coconut oil or olive oil
- 2-3 drops of vitamin E oil
- Optional: a few drops of your preferred essential oil for fragrance (such as lavender or tea tree)

Instructions:

- In a small bowl, combine the pure aloe vera gel and coconut oil or olive oil.
- Add 2-3 drops of vitamin E oil to the mixture.
- If desired, add a few drops of your chosen essential oil for a pleasant scent and added benefits.
- Stir all the ingredients together until well blended.
- Transfer the mixture to a clean, airtight container for storage.

How to use:

- Make sure your nails and cuticles are clean and dry.
- Take a small amount of the aloe vera gel cuticle oil on a cotton swab or your fingertips.
- Gently massage the oil into your cuticles and the surrounding nail area.
- Continue to massage for a few minutes to help the oil absorb.
- Repeat the process for each nail and cuticle.
- Use the cuticle oil regularly, ideally every night before bed, to keep your cuticles nourished and healthy.

Benefits:

- Aloe vera gel helps moisturize and soothe the cuticles, reducing dryness and promoting healthy nail growth.
- Coconut oil or olive oil provides nourishment and helps soften the cuticles, making them easier to push back or trim.
- Vitamin E oil provides antioxidant properties, protecting the cuticles from damage and promoting overall nail health.
- Essential oils can add a pleasant fragrance and provide additional benefits, such as antifungal or antibacterial properties.

Note: If you have any known allergies to the ingredients, it's important to avoid using this cuticle oil or do a patch test on a small area of your skin first to ensure you don't experience any adverse reactions.

Aloe Vera Gel After-Shave Lotion:

Creating your own aloe vera gel after-shave lotion is a great way to soothe and moisturize your skin after shaving. Here's a simple recipe for a DIY aloe vera gel after-shave lotion:

Ingredients:
- 1/4 cup of pure aloe vera gel
- 2 tablespoons of witch hazel
- 1 tablespoon of sweet almond oil or jojoba oil
- 5-10 drops of your preferred essential oil (such as lavender or tea tree)

Instructions:
- In a small bowl, combine the pure aloe vera gel, witch hazel, and sweet almond oil or jojoba oil.
- Add 5-10 drops of your chosen essential oil for fragrance and added benefits.
- Stir all the ingredients together until well blended.
- Transfer the mixture to a clean, airtight container for storage.

How to use:
- After shaving, rinse your skin with cold water and pat it dry with a towel.
- Take a small amount of the aloe vera gel after-shave lotion and apply it to the shaved areas of your face or body.
- Gently massage the lotion into your skin until it is fully absorbed.
- Allow the lotion to dry naturally before applying any additional products or clothing.

Benefits:
- Aloe vera gel helps soothe and calm the skin, reducing any irritation or redness caused by shaving.
- Witch hazel acts as an astringent, helping to tighten the pores and prevent ingrown hairs.
- Sweet almond oil or jojoba oil provide nourishment and moisturization to the skin, leaving it soft and smooth.
- Essential oils add a pleasant scent and offer additional benefits, such as antibacterial or anti-inflammatory properties.

Note: If you have any known allergies to the ingredients, it's important to avoid using this after-shave lotion or do a patch test on a small area of your skin first to ensure you don't experience any adverse reactions.

Aloe Vera Gel Bath Bombs:

Creating your own aloe vera gel bath bombs is a fun and luxurious way to enhance your bath time experience. Here's a simple recipe for DIY aloe vera gel bath bombs:

Ingredients:
- 1 cup baking soda
- 1/2 cup citric acid
- 1/2 cup cornstarch
- 1/4 cup Epsom salt
- 2 tablespoons aloe vera gel
- 1 tablespoon coconut oil or almond oil
- 1-2 teaspoons water

- 10-15 drops of your preferred essential oil
- Optional: dried flower petals or herbs for decoration

Instructions:
- In a mixing bowl, combine the baking soda, citric acid, cornstarch, and Epsom salt. Mix well to ensure even distribution of ingredients.
- In a separate small bowl, mix the aloe vera gel, coconut oil or almond oil, water, and essential oil together.
- Slowly pour the wet mixture into the dry mixture, stirring continuously to prevent fizzing.
- The mixture should hold its shape when squeezed together. If it's too dry, add a small amount of water at a time until the desired consistency is reached.
- Optional: Add dried flower petals or herbs into the mixture for decoration and added fragrance.
- Firmly pack the mixture into bath bomb molds or into your hands, pressing it tightly together.
- Let the bath bombs dry and harden in the molds for at least 24 hours. If you're using your hands, gently place them on a clean, dry surface and allow them to dry completely.
- Carefully remove the bath bombs from the molds or gently lift them off the surface if you formed them by hand.
- Store the bath bombs in an airtight container until ready to use.

How to use:
- Fill your bathtub with warm water.
- Drop one bath bomb into the water and watch it fizz and dissolve.
- Step into the bath and enjoy the soothing and moisturizing effects of the aloe vera gel bath bomb.
- Relax and soak for as long as desired.

Benefits:
- Aloe vera gel helps to moisturize and soothe the skin, leaving it feeling soft and hydrated.
- Baking soda and citric acid create a fizzy effect, making bath time more enjoyable.
- Epsom salt provides relaxation and may help relieve muscle tension.
- Essential oils add a pleasant scent and may offer additional benefits, depending on the chosen oil.

Note: If you have any known allergies to the ingredients, it's important to avoid using these bath bombs or do a patch test on a small area of your skin first to ensure you don't experience any adverse reactions. Exercise caution when using bath bombs with dried flower petals or herbs, as they may leave residue in the bathtub.

Aloe Vera Gel Face Scrub:

Creating your own aloe vera gel face scrub is a wonderful way to exfoliate and rejuvenate your skin. Here's a simple recipe for a DIY aloe vera gel face scrub:

Ingredients:

- 2 tablespoons of pure aloe vera gel
- 1 tablespoon of fine granulated sugar or brown sugar
- 1 teaspoon of lemon juice
- 1 teaspoon of coconut oil or olive oil
- Optional: a few drops of your preferred essential oil for fragrance (such as lavender or tea tree)

Instructions:

- In a small bowl, combine the pure aloe vera gel, granulated sugar, lemon juice, and coconut oil or olive oil.
- If desired, add a few drops of your chosen essential oil for a pleasant scent.
- Stir all the ingredients together until well mixed and the sugar is evenly distributed.
- Adjust the consistency by adding more sugar if you prefer a coarser scrub or more aloe vera gel if you prefer a gentler scrub.
- Transfer the mixture to a clean, airtight container for storage.

How to use:

- Wet your face with warm water to dampen the skin.
- Take a small amount of the aloe vera gel face scrub and gently massage it onto your face using circular motions.
- Pay extra attention to areas that need exfoliation, such as the T-zone or areas with dry patches.
- Avoid scrubbing too harshly, especially if you have sensitive skin.
- Rinse off the scrub thoroughly with warm water.
- Pat your face dry and follow with your regular skincare routine.

Benefits:

- Aloe vera gel helps to moisturize and soothe the skin, reducing any redness or irritation caused by exfoliation.
- Sugar acts as a natural exfoliant, helping to remove dead skin cells and unclog pores.
- Lemon juice provides a brightening effect and can help even out the skin tone.
- Coconut oil or olive oil moisturizes and nourishes the skin, leaving it soft and smooth.
- Essential oils add a pleasant fragrance and may provide additional benefits, depending on the chosen oil.

Note: If you have any known allergies to the ingredients, it's important to avoid using this face scrub or do a patch test on a small area of your skin first to ensure you don't experience any adverse reactions. Be gentle when using the scrub, especially if you have sensitive or acne-prone skin, as excessive scrubbing can cause irritation.

Aloe Vera Gel Hair Conditioner:

Creating your own aloe vera gel hair conditioner is a natural and nourishing way to hydrate and soften your hair. Here's a simple recipe for a DIY aloe vera gel hair conditioner:

Ingredients:

- 1/2 cup of pure aloe vera gel
- 2 tablespoons of coconut oil or olive oil
- 1 tablespoon of honey
- Optional: a few drops of your preferred essential oil for fragrance (such as lavender or rosemary)

Instructions:

- In a bowl, combine the pure aloe vera gel, coconut oil or olive oil, and honey.
- If desired, add a few drops of your chosen essential oil for a pleasant scent.
- Mix all the ingredients together until well blended.
- The mixture should have a smooth and creamy consistency.
- Transfer the conditioner to a clean, airtight container for storage.

How to use:

- After shampooing your hair, squeeze out any excess water.
- Take a small amount of the aloe vera gel hair conditioner and apply it to your hair, focusing on the mid-lengths and ends.
- Gently massage the conditioner into your hair, ensuring even distribution.
- Leave the conditioner on for a few minutes to allow it to penetrate the hair strands.
- Rinse your hair thoroughly with lukewarm water until the conditioner is completely washed out.
- Style your hair as desired.

Benefits:

- Aloe vera gel helps to moisturize and hydrate the hair, leaving it soft and manageable.
- Coconut oil or olive oil provides nourishment and helps to reduce frizz and enhance shine.
- Honey acts as a natural humectant, helping to lock in moisture and promote hair health.
- Essential oils add a pleasant fragrance and may provide additional benefits, such as promoting scalp health or stimulating hair growth.

Note: If you have any known allergies to the ingredients, it's important to avoid using this hair conditioner or do a patch test on a small area of your skin first to ensure you don't experience any adverse reactions. Adjust the amount of conditioner used based on the length and thickness of your hair. Use the conditioner 1-2 times per week or as needed to maintain soft and healthy hair.

Aloe Vera Gel Deodorant:

Creating your own aloe vera gel deodorant is a natural and effective way to stay fresh throughout the day. Here's a simple recipe for a DIY aloe vera gel deodorant:

Ingredients:
- 1/4 cup of pure aloe vera gel
- 1/4 cup of baking soda
- 1/4 cup of cornstarch or arrowroot powder
- 2 tablespoons of coconut oil
- Optional: a few drops of your preferred essential oil for fragrance (such as lavender or tea tree)

Instructions:
- In a mixing bowl, combine the pure aloe vera gel, baking soda, and cornstarch or arrowroot powder.
- Add the coconut oil to the mixture and stir until all the ingredients are well blended.
- If desired, add a few drops of your chosen essential oil for a pleasant scent.
- Adjust the consistency by adding more baking soda or cornstarch/arrowroot powder if needed to achieve a smooth, spreadable texture.
- Transfer the deodorant mixture to a clean, airtight container for storage.

How to use:
- Scoop a small amount of the aloe vera gel deodorant with your fingertips.
- Gently apply it to clean and dry underarms, massaging it into the skin until absorbed.
- Allow the deodorant to dry before putting on clothes.
- Reapply as needed throughout the day for maximum freshness.

Benefits:
- Aloe vera gel helps to soothe and moisturize the skin, reducing irritation and keeping the underarm area hydrated.
- Baking soda helps neutralize odor-causing bacteria, keeping you smelling fresh.
- Cornstarch or arrowroot powder helps absorb excess moisture, preventing wetness and discomfort.
- Coconut oil provides antimicrobial properties and helps the deodorant glide smoothly onto the skin.
- Essential oils add a pleasant fragrance and may offer additional antibacterial or antifungal benefits.

Note: If you have any known allergies to the ingredients, it's important to avoid using this deodorant or do a patch test on a small area of your skin first to ensure you don't experience any adverse reactions. Some individuals may be sensitive to baking soda, so monitor your skin for any signs of irritation. Store the deodorant in a cool, dry place.

Aloe Vera Gel Cooling Eye Mask:

Creating a DIY aloe vera gel cooling eye mask can provide soothing relief for tired, puffy eyes and help reduce under-eye circles. Here's a simple recipe for a homemade aloe vera gel cooling eye mask:

Ingredients:
- 2 tablespoons of pure aloe vera gel
- 1 tablespoon of cucumber juice (made by blending cucumber and straining the juice)
- 1-2 drops of chamomile essential oil (optional)

Instructions:
- In a small bowl, combine the pure aloe vera gel and cucumber juice.
- If desired, add 1-2 drops of chamomile essential oil for added relaxation.
- Stir the ingredients together until well mixed.
- Transfer the mixture to a clean, sealable container and store it in the refrigerator for a cooling effect.

How to use:
- Place the aloe vera gel cooling eye mask in the refrigerator for at least 30 minutes or until it's chilled.
- Gently cleanse your face and eyes to remove any makeup or dirt.
- Take out the chilled eye mask and apply it over your closed eyes, covering the entire eye area.
- Relax and leave the eye mask on for about 10-15 minutes.
- Afterward, remove the eye mask and discard any excess gel.
- Gently pat the area around your eyes with clean fingers to help the remaining gel absorb into the skin.
- You can follow up with an eye cream or moisturizer if desired.

Benefits:
- Aloe vera gel has soothing properties that can help reduce puffiness and calm tired eyes.
- Cucumber juice contains antioxidants and a cooling effect that can refresh the under-eye area.
- Chamomile essential oil, if used, can provide additional relaxation and soothing benefits.

Note: If you have any known allergies to the ingredients, it's important to avoid using this eye mask or do a patch test on a small area of your skin first to ensure you don't experience any adverse reactions. Avoid direct contact with the eyes and rinse immediately if any irritation occurs. The eye mask is for external use only.

Aloe Vera Gel Sunscreen:

Creating your own aloe vera gel sunscreen is a natural and moisturizing way to protect your skin from the sun's harmful rays. While aloe vera gel itself does not provide sufficient sun protection, you can combine it with other ingredients to make a DIY sunscreen. Here's a recipe for a homemade aloe vera gel sunscreen:

Ingredients:

- 1/4 cup of pure aloe vera gel
- 2 tablespoons of coconut oil
- 1 tablespoon of non-nano zinc oxide powder
- 1 tablespoon of shea butter
- Optional: a few drops of your preferred essential oil for fragrance (such as lavender or peppermint)

Instructions:

- In a heat-safe bowl, combine the pure aloe vera gel, coconut oil, and shea butter.
- Place the bowl over a pot of simmering water (creating a double boiler) and gently heat the mixture until the shea butter and coconut oil have melted completely.
- Once melted, remove the bowl from heat and let it cool for a few minutes.
- Add the non-nano zinc oxide powder to the mixture, stirring continuously to ensure it's well incorporated. Be cautious when working with zinc oxide to avoid inhaling the powder.
- If desired, add a few drops of your chosen essential oil for a pleasant scent.
- Transfer the sunscreen mixture to a clean, airtight container for storage.

How to use:

- Before sun exposure, apply a generous amount of the aloe vera gel sunscreen to all exposed areas of the skin.
- Gently massage the sunscreen into the skin until fully absorbed.
- Reapply every two hours or more frequently if sweating or after swimming.

Important notes:

- This DIY sunscreen is not water-resistant, so it's essential to reapply it regularly, especially after swimming or sweating.
- The non-nano zinc oxide provides physical sun protection by reflecting and scattering UV rays. However, it may leave a slight white cast on the skin.
- It's crucial to test the sunscreen on a small area of skin before using it extensively to ensure you don't experience any adverse reactions or allergies.
- This homemade sunscreen may have a lower sun protection factor (SPF) compared to commercial sunscreens. If you need higher SPF coverage, consider using additional protection or seeking commercial products.

Remember, protecting your skin from the sun is vital for overall skin health and to prevent sunburn, premature aging, and skin damage.

Aloe Vera Gel Body Wash

Creating your own aloe vera gel body wash is a great way to cleanse and nourish your skin.
Here's a simple recipe for a DIY aloe vera gel body wash:
Ingredients:

- 1 cup of liquid castile soap (unscented or your preferred scent)
- 1/4 cup of pure aloe vera gel
- 1 tablespoon of vegetable glycerin
- 1 tablespoon of sweet almond oil or jojoba oil
- Optional: a few drops of your preferred essential oil for fragrance (such as lavender or eucalyptus)

Instructions:

- In a mixing bowl, combine the liquid castile soap, pure aloe vera gel, vegetable glycerin, and sweet almond oil or jojoba oil.
- If desired, add a few drops of your chosen essential oil for a pleasant scent.
- Stir all the ingredients together until well blended.
- Transfer the body wash mixture to a clean, empty bottle or pump dispenser for easy use.

How to use:

- In the shower or bath, wet your body with warm water.
- Take a small amount of the aloe vera gel body wash in your hands or a loofah.
- Gently lather the body wash onto your skin, massaging in circular motions.
- Pay extra attention to areas that need cleansing or have dryness.
- Rinse off the body wash thoroughly with warm water.
- Pat your body dry and follow with your regular moisturizer if needed.

Benefits:

- Aloe vera gel helps to moisturize and soothe the skin, leaving it feeling soft and hydrated.
- Liquid castile soap is a gentle cleanser that effectively removes dirt and impurities without stripping the skin's natural oils.
- Vegetable glycerin provides additional moisture and helps maintain the skin's moisture balance.
- Sweet almond oil or jojoba oil nourishes and conditions the skin, promoting a healthy and radiant appearance.
- Essential oils add a pleasant fragrance and may offer additional benefits depending on the chosen oil.

Note: If you have any known allergies to the ingredients, it's important to avoid using this body wash or do a patch test on a small area of your skin first to ensure you don't experience any adverse reactions. Adjust the amount of body wash used based on personal preference. Store the body wash in a cool, dry place.

Aloe Vera Gel Hair Conditioner

Creating your own aloe vera gel hair conditioner is a natural and nourishing way to hydrate and soften your hair. Here's a simple recipe for a DIY aloe vera gel hair conditioner:

Ingredients:

- 1/4 cup of pure aloe vera gel
- 1/4 cup of coconut milk
- 1 tablespoon of honey
- 1 tablespoon of argan oil or jojoba oil
- Optional: a few drops of your preferred essential oil for fragrance (such as lavender or rosemary)

Instructions:

- In a blender or mixing bowl, combine the pure aloe vera gel, coconut milk, honey, and argan oil or jojoba oil.
- If desired, add a few drops of your chosen essential oil for a pleasant scent.
- Blend or whisk the ingredients together until you achieve a smooth and creamy consistency.
- Transfer the conditioner to a clean, airtight container for storage.

How to use:

- After shampooing your hair, squeeze out any excess water.
- Take a small amount of the aloe vera gel hair conditioner and apply it to your hair, focusing on the mid-lengths and ends.
- Gently massage the conditioner into your hair, ensuring even distribution.
- Leave the conditioner on for a few minutes to allow it to penetrate the hair strands.
- Rinse your hair thoroughly with lukewarm water until the conditioner is completely washed out.
- Style your hair as desired.

Benefits:

- Aloe vera gel helps to moisturize and hydrate the hair, leaving it soft and manageable.
- Coconut milk provides nourishment and helps to repair damaged hair.
- Honey acts as a natural humectant, helping to lock in moisture and promote hair health.
- Argan oil or jojoba oil provide additional hydration, softness, and shine to the hair.
- Essential oils add a pleasant fragrance and may provide additional benefits, such as promoting scalp health or stimulating hair growth.

Note: If you have any known allergies to the ingredients, it's important to avoid using this hair conditioner or do a patch test on a small area of your skin first to ensure you don't experience any adverse reactions. Adjust the amount of conditioner used based on the length and thickness of your hair. Use the conditioner 1-2 times per week or as needed to maintain soft and healthy hair. Store the conditioner in a cool, dry place.

Aloe Vera Gel Deodorant:

Creating your own aloe vera gel deodorant is a natural and effective way to stay fresh throughout the day. Here's a simple recipe for a DIY aloe vera gel deodorant:
Ingredients:

- 1/4 cup of pure aloe vera gel
- 2 tablespoons of baking soda
- 2 tablespoons of cornstarch or arrowroot powder
- 1 tablespoon of coconut oil
- Optional: a few drops of your preferred essential oil for fragrance (such as lavender or tea tree)

Instructions:

- In a mixing bowl, combine the pure aloe vera gel, baking soda, and cornstarch or arrowroot powder.
- Add the coconut oil to the mixture and stir until all the ingredients are well blended.
- If desired, add a few drops of your chosen essential oil for a pleasant scent.
- Adjust the consistency by adding more baking soda or cornstarch/arrowroot powder if needed to achieve a smooth, spreadable texture.
- Transfer the deodorant mixture to a clean, airtight container for storage.

How to use:

- Scoop a small amount of the aloe vera gel deodorant with your fingertips.
- Gently apply it to clean and dry underarms, massaging it into the skin until absorbed.
- Allow the deodorant to dry before putting on clothes.
- Reapply as needed throughout the day for maximum freshness.

Benefits:

- Aloe vera gel helps to soothe and moisturize the skin, reducing irritation and keeping the underarm area hydrated.
- Baking soda helps neutralize odor-causing bacteria, keeping you smelling fresh.
- Cornstarch or arrowroot powder helps absorb excess moisture, preventing wetness and discomfort.
- Coconut oil provides antimicrobial properties and helps the deodorant glide smoothly onto the skin.
- Essential oils add a pleasant fragrance and may offer additional antibacterial or antifungal benefits.

Note: If you have any known allergies to the ingredients, it's important to avoid using this deodorant or do a patch test on a small area of your skin first to ensure you don't experience any adverse reactions. Some individuals may be sensitive to baking soda, so monitor your skin for any signs of irritation. Store the deodorant in a cool, dry place.

Aloe Vera Gel Cooling Eye Mask:

Creating a DIY aloe vera gel cooling eye mask is a simple and effective way to soothe tired eyes, reduce puffiness, and relax. Here's a step-by-step guide on how to make an aloe vera gel cooling eye mask:

Materials:
- Aloe vera gel
- Small bowl
- Cotton rounds or cotton pads
- Plastic wrap or a small plastic bag
- Refrigerator

Instructions:
- Start by placing the aloe vera gel in a small bowl. Ensure that the gel is pure and free from added colors or fragrances.
- Take the cotton rounds or cotton pads and dip them into the aloe vera gel, saturating them completely.
- Squeeze out any excess gel from the cotton rounds, but make sure they are still moist.
- Place the moistened cotton rounds in a plastic bag or wrap them in plastic wrap to keep them from drying out.
- Put the bag or wrapped cotton rounds in the refrigerator and let them cool for at least 30 minutes.
- Once chilled, remove the cotton rounds from the bag or plastic wrap.
- Lie down in a comfortable position and place the chilled cotton rounds over your closed eyes, ensuring that they cover the entire eye area.
- Relax and leave the cooling eye mask on for about 10-15 minutes.
- Afterward, remove the cotton rounds and discard them.
- Gently massage the area around your eyes with clean fingertips to help the remaining aloe vera gel absorb into the skin.
- If desired, follow up with an eye cream or moisturizer.

Benefits:
- Aloe vera gel has soothing properties that can help reduce puffiness, calm irritation, and provide a cooling sensation to the eyes.
- The cooling effect helps alleviate tiredness and can be refreshing after a long day or exposure to screen time.
- Aloe vera gel contains hydrating properties that can help moisturize the delicate skin around the eyes.

Note: It's essential to ensure the aloe vera gel is pure and free from any added ingredients that may cause irritation. Avoid placing the cooling eye mask directly on open wounds, irritated skin, or directly on the eyes. If you experience any discomfort or adverse reactions, discontinue use.

Aloe Vera Gel Sunscreen:

Creating your own aloe vera gel sunscreen is a natural and moisturizing way to protect your skin from the sun's harmful rays. However, it's important to note that aloe vera gel alone does not provide sufficient sun protection. You can combine it with other ingredients to make a DIY sunscreen. Here's a recipe for a homemade aloe vera gel sunscreen:

Ingredients:

- 1/4 cup of pure aloe vera gel
- 2 tablespoons of shea butter
- 1 tablespoon of coconut oil
- 1 tablespoon of non-nano zinc oxide powder
- Optional: a few drops of your preferred essential oil for fragrance (such as lavender or peppermint)

Instructions:

- In a heat-safe bowl, combine the pure aloe vera gel, shea butter, and coconut oil.
- Place the bowl over a pot of simmering water (creating a double boiler) and gently heat the mixture until the shea butter and coconut oil have melted completely.
- Once melted, remove the bowl from heat and let it cool for a few minutes.
- Add the non-nano zinc oxide powder to the mixture, stirring continuously to ensure it's well incorporated. Be cautious when working with zinc oxide to avoid inhaling the powder.
- If desired, add a few drops of your chosen essential oil for a pleasant scent.
- Transfer the sunscreen mixture to a clean, airtight container for storage.

How to use:

- Before sun exposure, apply a generous amount of the aloe vera gel sunscreen to all exposed areas of the skin.
- Gently massage the sunscreen into the skin until fully absorbed.
- Reapply every two hours or more frequently if sweating or after swimming.

Important notes:

- The non-nano zinc oxide provides physical sun protection by reflecting and scattering UV rays. However, it may leave a slight white cast on the skin.
- It's crucial to test the sunscreen on a small area of skin before using it extensively to ensure you don't experience any adverse reactions or allergies.
- This homemade sunscreen may have a lower sun protection factor (SPF) compared to commercial sunscreens. If you need higher SPF coverage, consider using additional protection or seeking commercial products.

Remember, protecting your skin from the sun is vital for overall skin health and to prevent sunburn, premature aging, and skin damage. It's always a good idea to consult with a dermatologist or medical professional for personalized advice on sun protection and suitable sunscreen options for your specific needs.

Aloe Vera Gel Bath Soak:

Creating a soothing and relaxing aloe vera gel bath soak can be a wonderful way to pamper yourself and nourish your skin. Here's a simple recipe for a DIY aloe vera gel bath soak:

Ingredients:

- 1 cup of Epsom salt
- 1/2 cup of baking soda
- 1/4 cup of pure aloe vera gel
- Optional: a few drops of your preferred essential oil for fragrance (such as lavender or chamomile)

Instructions:

- In a mixing bowl, combine the Epsom salt and baking soda.
- Add the pure aloe vera gel to the mixture and stir until it is well incorporated.
- If desired, add a few drops of your chosen essential oil for a pleasant scent and extra relaxation.
- Mix all the ingredients thoroughly to ensure they are evenly distributed.

How to use:

- Fill your bathtub with warm water.
- Add the aloe vera gel bath soak mixture to the running water as the tub fills.
- Stir the water with your hand to help dissolve the ingredients.
- Once the bath is filled, soak in the tub for at least 20 minutes, allowing your body to relax and absorb the benefits of the aloe vera gel and Epsom salt.
- Gently rinse your body with warm water after the soak to remove any residue.
- Pat your skin dry and follow with your preferred moisturizer if desired.

Benefits:

- Epsom salt is known for its soothing and muscle-relaxing properties. It can help reduce tension, promote relaxation, and relieve soreness.
- Baking soda may help soften the water and soothe the skin, leaving it feeling refreshed.
- Aloe vera gel helps moisturize and nourish the skin, leaving it soft and hydrated.
- Essential oils add a pleasant fragrance and can enhance the overall relaxation experience.

Note: If you have any known allergies to the ingredients, it's important to avoid using this bath soak or do a patch test on a small area of your skin first to ensure you don't experience any adverse reactions. Adjust the amount of bath soak used based on personal preference. Store any remaining bath soak mixture in a cool, dry place.

Aloe Vera Gel Body Scrub:

Creating a homemade aloe vera gel body scrub is a great way to exfoliate and rejuvenate your skin. Here's a simple recipe for a DIY aloe vera gel body scrub:

Ingredients:
- 1/2 cup of granulated sugar (or salt for a coarser scrub)
- 1/4 cup of pure aloe vera gel
- 2 tablespoons of coconut oil (melted)
- Optional: a few drops of your preferred essential oil for fragrance (such as citrus or peppermint)

Instructions:
- In a mixing bowl, combine the granulated sugar (or salt) and pure aloe vera gel.
- Add the melted coconut oil to the mixture and stir until it forms a paste-like consistency.
- If desired, add a few drops of your chosen essential oil for a pleasant scent and extra relaxation.
- Mix all the ingredients thoroughly to ensure they are well blended.

How to use:
- Begin by wetting your skin in the shower or bath.
- Take a small amount of the aloe vera gel body scrub and gently massage it onto your body in circular motions, focusing on areas that need exfoliation or extra care.
- Continue massaging for a few minutes, allowing the scrub to slough away dead skin cells and moisturize the skin.
- Rinse off the scrub with warm water.
- Follow up with your regular shower routine or apply a moisturizer to seal in the hydration.

Benefits:
- Sugar or salt acts as a natural exfoliant, helping to remove dead skin cells and promote smoother, softer skin.
- Aloe vera gel provides hydration and nourishment to the skin, leaving it moisturized and refreshed.
- Coconut oil helps to moisturize and soften the skin, leaving it feeling smooth and supple.
- Essential oils add a pleasant fragrance and may offer additional benefits, such as invigorating or calming effects.

Note: If you have any known allergies to the ingredients, it's important to avoid using this body scrub or do a patch test on a small area of your skin first to ensure you don't experience any adverse reactions. Adjust the amount of body scrub used based on personal preference. Use gentle pressure when scrubbing to avoid irritating the skin. Store any remaining scrub in an airtight container in a cool, dry place.

Aloe Vera Gel Soothing Gel for Bug Bites:

Creating a homemade aloe vera gel soothing gel for bug bites is a natural and gentle way to alleviate itchiness, reduce inflammation, and promote healing. Here's a simple recipe for a DIY aloe vera gel soothing gel for bug bites:

Ingredients:
- 2 tablespoons of pure aloe vera gel
- 1 teaspoon of witch hazel
- 1 teaspoon of coconut oil (melted)
- Optional: a few drops of lavender essential oil (known for its soothing properties)

Instructions:
- In a small bowl, combine the pure aloe vera gel, witch hazel, and melted coconut oil.
- Stir the mixture thoroughly to ensure all the ingredients are well blended.
- If desired, add a few drops of lavender essential oil for its additional calming and soothing effects.
- Mix well to incorporate the essential oil into the gel.

How to use:
- Clean the affected area with mild soap and water.
- Apply a small amount of the aloe vera gel soothing gel to the bug bite.
- Gently massage the gel into the skin, ensuring it covers the entire bite area.
- Allow the gel to absorb into the skin.
- Repeat the application as needed to soothe itchiness and discomfort.

Benefits:
- Aloe vera gel contains anti-inflammatory properties that can help reduce redness, swelling, and itching caused by bug bites.
- Witch hazel is known for its astringent and soothing properties, which can help alleviate irritation and inflammation.
- Coconut oil helps moisturize and nourish the skin, promoting healing.
- Lavender essential oil has calming and soothing effects that may further help relieve itchiness and discomfort.

Note: It's important to ensure the aloe vera gel is pure and free from any added ingredients that may cause irritation. If you have any known allergies to the ingredients, it's recommended to do a patch test on a small area of your skin first to ensure you don't experience any adverse reactions. If you have severe reactions to bug bites or if symptoms persist, it's advisable to consult a healthcare professional.

Aloe Vera Gel Cooling Foot Spray:

Creating a DIY aloe vera gel cooling foot spray can provide a refreshing and soothing sensation for tired, hot, or achy feet. Here's a simple recipe for an aloe vera gel cooling foot spray:

Ingredients:
- 1/4 cup of pure aloe vera gel
- 1/4 cup of witch hazel
- 10 drops of peppermint essential oil
- 5 drops of tea tree essential oil
- Distilled water
- Spray bottle

Instructions:
- In a small bowl, combine the pure aloe vera gel, witch hazel, peppermint essential oil, and tea tree essential oil.
- Mix the ingredients thoroughly until they are well blended.
- Pour the mixture into a spray bottle.
- Fill the remaining space in the bottle with distilled water, leaving a little room at the top for shaking.
- Close the spray bottle tightly and shake well to combine all the ingredients.

How to use:
- Shake the bottle before each use to ensure the ingredients are well mixed.
- Spray the cooling foot spray directly onto your feet, targeting the soles, heels, and any areas that feel hot or tired.
- Gently massage the spray into your feet to enhance the cooling sensation.
- Allow the spray to dry naturally.

Benefits:
- Aloe vera gel provides a cooling and soothing effect, helping to reduce heat and relieve discomfort in the feet.
- Witch hazel has a refreshing and astringent effect that can help reduce swelling and inflammation.
- Peppermint essential oil provides a cooling sensation and has a refreshing aroma that can help revive tired feet.
- Tea tree essential oil has natural antibacterial properties that can help keep the feet fresh and clean.

Note: If you have any known allergies to the ingredients, it's recommended to do a patch test on a small area of your skin first to ensure you don't experience any adverse reactions. Avoid spraying the cooling foot spray on open wounds or broken skin. If you experience any discomfort or irritation, discontinue use.

Aloe Vera Gel Hand Cream:

Creating a homemade aloe vera gel hand cream is a great way to moisturize and nourish your hands, especially if they feel dry or rough. Here's a simple recipe for a DIY aloe vera gel hand cream:

Ingredients:

- 1/4 cup of pure aloe vera gel
- 2 tablespoons of shea butter
- 1 tablespoon of coconut oil
- 1 teaspoon of vitamin E oil
- Optional: a few drops of your preferred essential oil for fragrance (such as lavender or citrus)

Instructions:

- In a heat-safe bowl, combine the pure aloe vera gel, shea butter, and coconut oil.
- Place the bowl over a pot of simmering water (creating a double boiler) and gently heat the mixture until the shea butter and coconut oil have melted completely.
- Once melted, remove the bowl from heat and let it cool for a few minutes.
- Add the vitamin E oil to the mixture, along with a few drops of your chosen essential oil for fragrance if desired.
- Stir the mixture well to ensure all the ingredients are combined.
- Transfer the hand cream mixture to a clean, airtight container for storage.

How to use:

- Take a small amount of the hand cream and massage it into your hands.
- Pay extra attention to dry or rough areas, such as the knuckles or cuticles.
- Allow the cream to absorb into your skin.
- Reapply as needed, especially after washing your hands or when your skin feels dry.

Benefits:

- Aloe vera gel provides hydration and nourishment to the skin, leaving your hands moisturized and soft.
- Shea butter is rich in vitamins and fatty acids that help moisturize and protect the skin, promoting its smoothness and elasticity.
- Coconut oil is deeply moisturizing and has antimicrobial properties that can help prevent dryness and protect against germs.
- Vitamin E oil is an antioxidant that can help nourish and protect the skin from environmental damage.

Note: If you have any known allergies to the ingredients, it's important to avoid using this hand cream or do a patch test on a small area of your skin first to ensure you don't experience any adverse reactions. Adjust the amount of hand cream used based on personal preference. Store the hand cream in a cool, dry place.

Aloe Vera Gel Leave-In Conditioner:

Creating a homemade aloe vera gel leave-in conditioner is an excellent way to hydrate and nourish your hair, leaving it smooth, soft, and manageable. Here's a simple recipe for a DIY aloe vera gel leave-in conditioner:

Ingredients:
- 1/2 cup of pure aloe vera gel
- 1 tablespoon of vegetable glycerin
- 1 tablespoon of jojoba oil (or your preferred carrier oil)
- 5-10 drops of your preferred essential oil for fragrance (optional)

Instructions:
- In a mixing bowl, combine the pure aloe vera gel, vegetable glycerin, and jojoba oil.
- If desired, add a few drops of your chosen essential oil for a pleasant fragrance and added benefits.
- Mix all the ingredients thoroughly until well blended.

How to use:
- Wash your hair as usual and towel-dry until damp.
- Take a small amount of the aloe vera gel leave-in conditioner and rub it between your palms.
- Apply the conditioner evenly throughout your hair, focusing on the mid-lengths and ends.
- Gently comb or finger-style your hair to distribute the conditioner.
- Style your hair as desired. There's no need to rinse out the conditioner.

Benefits:
- Aloe vera gel helps to moisturize the hair, promoting hydration and reducing frizz.
- Vegetable glycerin acts as a humectant, attracting moisture to the hair and keeping it hydrated.
- Jojoba oil nourishes and conditions the hair, adding shine and improving manageability.
- Essential oils provide a pleasant scent and may offer additional benefits depending on the chosen oil.

Note: If you have any known allergies to the ingredients, it's important to avoid using this leave-in conditioner or do a patch test on a small area of your skin first to ensure you don't experience any adverse reactions. Adjust the amount of leave-in conditioner used based on your hair length and thickness. Store any remaining conditioner in a cool, dry place.

Aloe Vera Gel Body Mist:

Creating a homemade aloe vera gel body mist is a wonderful way to refresh and hydrate your skin, leaving it feeling cool and revitalized. Here's a simple recipe for a DIY aloe vera gel body mist:

Ingredients:
- 1/2 cup of pure aloe vera gel
- 1 cup of distilled water

- 1-2 tablespoons of witch hazel
- Optional: a few drops of your preferred essential oil for fragrance (such as lavender or citrus)

Instructions:

In a spray bottle, combine the pure aloe vera gel, distilled water, and witch hazel.

If desired, add a few drops of your chosen essential oil for a pleasant scent and added benefits.

Close the spray bottle tightly and shake well to ensure all the ingredients are thoroughly mixed.

How to use:

Shake the bottle before each use to distribute the ingredients evenly.

Hold the bottle about 6-8 inches away from your body.

Spray the mist generously over your body, avoiding the face and eyes.

Allow the mist to air dry or gently pat it into your skin.

Benefits:

- Aloe vera gel provides a cooling and soothing effect on the skin, making it a perfect ingredient for a refreshing body mist.
- Distilled water helps to hydrate and refresh the skin, especially during hot weather or when your skin feels dry.
- Witch hazel has astringent properties that can help tighten the pores and provide a subtle toning effect.
- Essential oils add a pleasant fragrance and may offer additional benefits depending on the chosen oil.

Note: If you have any known allergies to the ingredients, it's important to avoid using this body mist or do a patch test on a small area of your skin first to ensure you don't experience any adverse reactions. Avoid spraying the mist on broken or irritated skin. Discontinue use if any irritation occurs. Store the body mist in a cool, dry place.